DATE DUE

10/14/4	

TO RENEW:
760-744-1150 X 8113

PRINTED IN U.S.A.

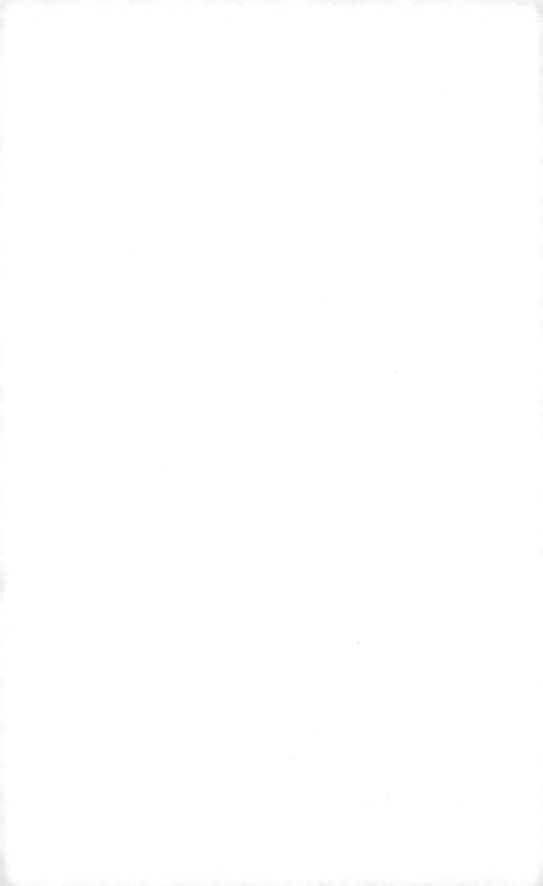

What's Wrong with Fat?

What's Wrong with Fat?

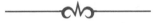

Abigail C. Saguy

OXFORD
UNIVERSITY PRESS

OXFORD
UNIVERSITY PRESS

Oxford University Press is a department of the
University of Oxford. It furthers the University's objective
of excellence in research, scholarship, and education
by publishing worldwide

Oxford   New York

Auckland   Cape Town   Dar es Salaam   Hong Kong   Karachi
Kuala Lumpur   Madrid   Melbourne   Mexico City   Nairobi
New Delhi   Shanghai   Taipei   Toronto

With offices in

Argentina   Austria   Brazil   Chile   Czech Republic   France   Greece
Guatemala   Hungary   Italy   Japan   Poland   Portugal   Singapore
South Korea   Switzerland   Thailand   Turkey   Ukraine   Vietnam

Oxford is a registered trademark of Oxford University Press
in the UK and certain other countries

Published in the United States of America by
Oxford University Press
198 Madison Avenue, New York, New York 10016

Library of Congress Cataloging-in-Publication Data
Saguy, Abigail C.
What's wrong with fat? / Abigail C. Saguy.
p.   cm.
Includes bibliographical references and index.
ISBN 978-0-19-985708-1 (alk. paper)
1. Obesity—Social aspects.   I. Title.
RA645.O23S24   2013
616.3'98—dc23   2012019331

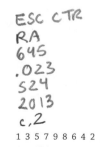
1 3 5 7 9 8 6 4 2

Printed in the United States of America
on acid-free paper

For Dotan

CONTENTS

ACKNOWLEDGMENTS

This project began on a snowy day in January 2001 in a seminar room at Yale University. I was sitting around a table with several thirty-something–year-old political scientists, sociologists, and economists who were, like me, enrolled in a two-year postdoctoral program in health policy, sponsored by the Robert Wood Johnson Foundation (RWJF). We were debating why obesity was not on the public agenda, despite the presumed fact that "overweight" and "obesity" were responsible for almost as many premature deaths as cigarette smoking.[1] This discussion launched me on a decade of research on the scientific debates and news media representation of "obesity," political mobilizing over fat rights, and the material implications of different "fat frames." I benefited from discussions with RWJF faculty and postdocs at Yale, University of California–Berkeley, and University of Michigan and from my own and earlier cohorts, including Eric Oliver, Taeku Lee, Rogan Kersh, Ted Marmor, Kimberly DaCosta, Evan Lieberman, John Cawley, Vincent Hutchings, Ann Keller, Bradley Herring, Karl Kronebusch, Mark Suchman, and Gary McKissick. I am especially grateful for the encouragement and invaluable feedback Mark Schlesinger provided at early stages of this research.

The Fund for the Advancement of the Discipline (cosponsored by the American Sociological Association and the National Science Foundation); the Partner University Fund, a program of FACE; and the Center for Advanced Studies in the Behavioral Sciences (CASBS) at Stanford University provided additional financial support. I also received funding from the UCLA Department of Sociology and several UCLA centers and organizations—including the Graduate Research Mentorship Program, the Center for American Politics and Public Policy, the Institute for Society and Genetics, the Center for the Study of Women, and the Academic Senate.

I could not have conducted this research were it not for all of the people who agreed to be interviewed and took the time to answer my questions. Marilyn Wann, Deb Burgard, and Bill Fabrey deserve special thanks for the countless insights they shared over the years. I also learned much from informal discussions and e-mail exchanges with Katherine Flegal, Linda Bacon, and Charlotte Cooper. Much of the data and parts of the argument presented here were first developed in collaborations for journal articles with exceptional graduate student research assistants, including Kjerstin Gruys, David Frederick, Rene Almeling, Kevin Riley, Anna Ward, and Shanna Gong. This book also benefited from outstanding research assistance from several undergraduate and graduate students, including Isabelle Huguet Lee, Erika Hernandez, Roxana Ghashghaei, Jeanine Yang, Rachel Berger, Amberia Allen, Nicole Iturriaga, Ruth Do, Michael Chow, Rebecca DiBennardo, and Jen Morony.

In 2003, I read and commented on a draft of Paul Campos's *Obesity Myth*, beginning a dialogue that would continue over years. Our ongoing conversation has deeply shaped this project. At a visit to Princeton's sociology department, where I presented a working paper from this project, one of my former graduate student mentors, Paul DiMaggio, encouraged me to develop the idea of a "fat field." Marion Fourcade later pushed me along these same lines, when we were both research fellows at CASBS from 2008 to 2009. This resulted in a PowerPoint presentation to my CASBS cohort, which provided the basis for the discussion of the fat field in chapter 2. Comments from Lynne Gerber and Adam Isaiah Green helped me to better hone in on my use of this concept. Adam Isaiah Green also provided valuable feedback on the introduction and conclusion; Lynne Gerber read and commented on the entire manuscript.

During my year at the idyllic CASBS at Stanford University, I had the opportunity to exchange ideas with thoughtful scholars working in a range of different academic disciplines at the center or at Stanford University. Discussions with Marion Fourcade, Chandra Mukerji, Deborah Rhode, Kieran Healy, Steven Epstein, Philip Howard, Rose McDermott, France Winddance Twine, Nancy Cott, Hazel Markus, John Lucy, Karen Knorr, Andrei Markovits, Glenn Adams, Kate Stovell, and Claude Steele all shaped this book. I also benefited from a CASBS workshop on writing for a general audience. My agent, Jill Marsal, provided valuable guidance in conceptualizing the book project in the early stages and in pitching it to publishers. My Oxford University Press editor, James Cook, offered useful editorial suggestions. I received two rounds of valuable feedback from anonymous peer reviewers for Oxford University Press. Gwen Colvin and Suzanne Austin copyedited the final manuscript. I have also benefited from comments received from several nonacademic friends, including Charlotte Elkin, Sarah Istwany, Kate Watkins, and Sherri Zigman.

I presented papers from this project at several meetings of the American Sociological Association and at meetings of the Law and Society Association. I presented to departmental workshops across the country, including the Yale Center for Eating and Weight Disorders workshop, Princeton University Sociology, UC San Diego Sociology (several times), UC Irvine Sociology, UC Berkeley Sociology (twice), UC Berkeley Center for the Study of Law and

Society, UC Santa Barbara Sociology, Northwestern Sociology, Northwestern Program in Comparative-Historical Social Science, RAND, the University of Texas– Austin Sociology, University of Colorado–Boulder Law School and Sociology Department, and the Siciliano Forum at the University of Utah. Abroad, I presented this work at the "Eurobese Workshop" in Chatilly, France; a workshop on the body, moral discourses, and society at the Van Leer Institute in Jerusalem; a Culture and Power conference in Oslo; the Institut National de la Recherche Agronomique in Paris, France; the University of Toulouse II–Le Mirail; l'Ecole des Hautes Etudes en Sciences Sociales in Paris; and the University of Paris VII. Members of these various audiences had thoughtful reactions. I am especially grateful for feedback from Anna Kirkland, Christine Williams, Kathleen LeBesco, John Evans, Sigal Gooldin, Henri Bergeron, Patrick Castel, Thibaut de Saint Pol, Jean Pierre Poulain, Barry Glassner, Paul Lichterman, Nina Eliasoph, Brian Finch, Iddo Tavery, Ted Chiricos, Peer Fiss, James Mahoney, Monica Prasad, Bruce Western, Viviana Zelizer, Anne Swidler, Michael Hout, Deana Rohlinger, Barbara Katz Rothman, Linda Blum, Michèle Lamont, Rodney Benson, Shari Dworkin, Wendy Griswold, Paul McAuley, Muriel Darmon, Joshua Gamson, and Nicola Beisel.

While most of the analysis in this book is new, parts of several chapters were published as "Morality and Health: News Media Constructions of Overweight and Eating Disorders," *Social Problems* 57, no 2 (2010): 231–50 (coauthored with Kjerstin Gruys); "Social Problem Construction and National Context: News Reporting on 'Overweight' and 'Obesity' in the U.S. and France," *Social Problems* 57, no. 4 (2010): 586–610 (coauthored with Kjerstin Gruys and Shanna Gong); "Fat in the Fire? Science, the News Media, and the 'Obesity Epidemic,'" *Sociological Forum* 23, no. 1 (2008): 53–83 (coauthored with Rene Almeling); "Weighing Both Sides: Morality, Mortality and Framing Contests over Obesity," *Journal of Health Politics, Policy, and Law* 30, no. 5 (2005): 869–921 (coauthored with Kevin W. Riley); and "Coming Out as Fat: Rethinking Stigma," *Social Psychology Quarterly* 74, no. 1 (2011): 53–75 (coauthored with Anna Ward).

UCLA has provided a stimulating intellectual community in which to develop my ideas. I presented this work to several UCLA groups, including the Comparative Historical Workshop in Sociology, the Law School, the Center for the Study of Women, and the Institute for Society and Genetics. I am grateful for collegial support and stimulating discussions with my UCLA colleagues, especially William Roy, Stefan Timmermans, Traci Mann, Mignon Moore, Megan Sweeney, Andrea Ghez, Kathleen McHugh, Christine Littleton, Aziza Khazzoom, Steve Clayman, Nicky Hart, Ike Grusky, Gail Kligman, Gabriel Rossman, Allison Hoffman, Aaron Panofsky, Elizabeth Frankenberg, Ruth Milkman, Judith Seltzer, David Lopez, Roger Waldinger, and Scott Waugh.

Edward Walker and former UCLA student Rene Almeling provided valuable comments on several book chapters. A graduate seminar I taught on gender and the body during the fall of 2011 provided an engaging intellectual forum in which to develop many of the ideas in this book; students in this class provided useful feedback on the introduction and chapter 2. Lianna Hart offered extremely valuable comments on several book chapters.

I had the good fortune to be a part of a UCLA-based writing group during the two years that I wrote and rewrote this book manuscript. During this time, I received invaluable insights from each member of this group, including Hannah Landecker, Juliet Williams, Lieba Faier, Jessica Cattelino, and Purnima Mankekar. This group was intellectual community at its best: challenging yet supportive and a source of creativity and renewed excitement. Members of this writing group pushed me to include illustrations to help explain the central concept of framing. Ian Patrick produced elegant and clever illustrations that greatly surpassed my expectations.

My mother, Rita Smith, a fan of Weight Watchers and Jane Brody's columns, took a while to understand the central goals of this research project and the perspective underlying it. Her skepticism helped me better articulate my argument. She also took it upon herself to forward me every *New York Times* discussion related to body weight and diet. My father, Charles W. Smith, is one of the best sociologists I know and has shaped me in more ways than I myself could possibly realize, as he himself likes to remind me from time to time.

I was pregnant with my daughter, Claire, when I began research on this book; my son, Jonah, was born two and a half years later. I have thus been working on this project for their entire lives. Recently Claire and Jonah have actively engaged in discussions with me that inform this book. I am deeply grateful to have the opportunity to be their mother and for the sweetness and meaning they add to my life. Finally, my husband, Dotan, makes it all possible. He is a truly egalitarian partner who has always valued my happiness and success as much as his own. His active engagement in our family has allowed me to throw myself into my research and writing and present my findings across the country and abroad, while raising two young children. He has embraced this research project as his own, always on the lookout for relevant news articles and ready with suggestions for catchy book titles and covers. He is my biggest fan, telling anyone who will listen about this research and why it is important. I dedicate this book to him.

health; the beauty frame, in which fatness is seen as beautiful; and a fat rights frame, according to which weight-based discrimination, not fatness itself, is the problem.[1]

Table 2.1 provides an overview of the six problem frames discussed in this chapter, showing what each frame implies about: *what* (if anything) is wrong with fatness, what should be done, associated analogies, key supporters, the gender of proponents, and the *master frame* on which the particular problem frame draws.[2] The equal rights master frame is a classic example of a master frame. The U.S. civil rights movement, women's movement, gay rights movement, and disability movement all draw on an "equal rights" master frame, which first became prominent in the southern black freedom movement of the 1950s.[3] Indeed, a small but vocal fat rights movement is currently trying to extend the equal rights master frame to body size by likening weight-based discrimination to racial, gender, or sexual orientation discrimination. In contrast, as we will see, the medical, public health crisis, and health at every size frames all draw on a master frame of health. These frames are not exhaustive; one could identify additional problem frames and subframes.[4] Yet these six frames capture many of the important cleavages in contemporary debates over fatness.

CREDIBILITY STRUGGLES IN THE FAT FIELD

Presenting these different frames in a neat five-by-five table obscures the fact that they are not competing on an equal playing field. The frames, and the people and institutions advancing them, vary widely in their influence and power. To illustrate this, it is helpful to draw upon Bourdieu's concept of *field*, a semiautonomous social space with its own rules such as the political, academic, artistic, and journalistic fields. People and institutions compete for distinction and influence within specific fields, based on that field's rules and associated forms of capital. In addition to *economic capital*, which refers to monetary resources, there is *symbolic capital*, which is based on honor, prestige, or recognition. Two specific forms of symbolic capital include *social capital*, or the actual or potential resources linked to social networks, and *cultural capital*, the knowledge, skills (including "soft skills"), and education that give a person advantages in a given society.[5] Specific institutions, groups, and individuals vary in the amount and kind of capital they possess, providing incentives either to shore up or to challenge the rules governing who has influence and power within a field. For instance, when U.S. civil rights and women's groups challenged the role of "old boys' networks" to confer status and privilege, they contested the legitimacy of a

Table 2.1

	Immorality	Medical	Public Health Crisis	Health at Every Size	Beauty	Fat Rights
What's wrong with fat?	Fat is evidence of sloth and gluttony, a *moral* problem.	Excess weight/fat is a *medical* problem.	Increasing population weights is a *public health crisis*.	The focus on weight loss and dieting are *health* problems.	Tendency to equate thinness with beauty is an *aesthetic* problem.	Weight-based discrimination is a *social justice* problem.
What should be done?	People need to exercise moral restraint.	We need to find medical means to help individuals lose weight.	We need to reduce BMI at the population level.	People of all sizes should learn to eat in response to internal cues and to exercise for its intrinsic benefits.	Fat should be seen as beautiful.	We need to combat fat bias and weight-based discrimination in employment, public spaces, health care, and elsewhere.
Master frame	Sin	Health	Health, Economic	Health	Aesthetics	Equal Rights
Analogies	Sexual immorality	Cancer, smoking	Epidemic, smoking	Yellow teeth, baldness	Clear complexion	Race, gender, sexual orientation, disability
Proponents	Religious authorities	Bariatric doctors, medical journals	CDC, WHO, IASO, NAASO, IOTF, Hoffman-La Roche, commercial weight-loss companies	ASDAH, NAAFA	NAAFA, fat admirers	Fat rights movement and organizations
Gender of proponents	Male dominated	Male dominated	Male dominated	Female dominated	Male dominated	Female dominated

specific form of social capital that favors white men and disadvantages women and ethnic minorities.

Building on Bourdieu's concept of field, we can conceptualize a *fat field,* in which the meaning of fat is contested. Organized around a topic, rather than a single institution, a fat field can nonetheless be conceptualized as a semiautonomous field with its own rules and forms of relevant capital. Figure 2.1, is a visual representation of some of the key players in the fat field, mapped on a matrix, in which the y-axis represents the volume of capital possessed by each institution, company, industry, or group of individuals and the x-axis shows the relative balance between cultural and economic power or capital. In a traditional matrix analysis, the position of actors would be determined based on calculations of actual capital.[6] In contrast, the figure should be taken as sensitizing, rather than as empirically exact. It provides a visual representation of the relative power of key interest groups that is grounded in my knowledge of how these different groups vary by their economic and cultural capital. In the interest of simplicity and readability, this figure only shows a few key players who feature prominently in this chapter and makes no claims to be exhaustive. Those higher on the vertical axis possess more capital of any kind. Those further to the left possess a greater proportion of symbolic, compared to economic, capital. In contrast, those further to the right possess a greater proportion of economic, relative to symbolic, capital.

The International Obesity Task Force (IOTF), International Association for the Study of Obesity (IASO), and National American Association for the Study of Obesity (NAASO), which have been at the forefront of promoting a public health crisis frame, are featured high on this graph and toward the middle, reflecting the high volume of both economic and symbolic capital they possess. Generous funding from pharmaceutical companies that produce weight-loss products has provided high levels of economic capital to these groups, while their ability to recruit doctors and researchers with prestigious educational credentials has given them high levels of symbolic capital as well.[7] The placement of the pharmaceutical company Hoffman-La Roche, who has directly promoted a public health crisis frame, at the top right-hand corner reflects its high levels of mostly economic capital, valued in 2007 at $153.55 billion.[8] The Centers for Disease Control and Prevention (CDC), World Health Organization (WHO), and National Institutes of Health (NIH), who have promoted a public health crisis frame, are on the top left because they have high levels of capital that is weighted more heavily toward symbolic capital.

Weight Watchers is shown close to the center line in the top right-hand corner, reflecting both its considerable economic capital ($1.4 billion in revenue and $177 million in net income in 2009) and the symbolic capital

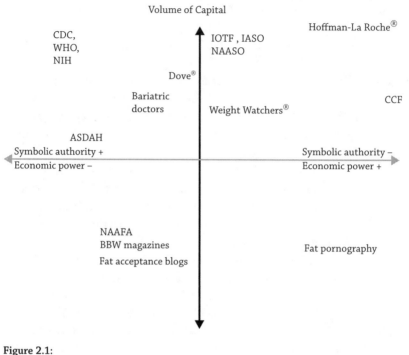

Figure 2.1:
The Fat Field

it enjoys due to its status as a more "healthy"/medically sound approach to weight loss, compared to the various fad diets available. Its main competitors, not shown in the figure, include Nestle, the company that owns Jenny Craig and Lean Cuisine brands, NutriSystem, and LA Weight Loss. In Britain, Slimming World is bigger than Weight Watchers.[9] The Center for Consumer Freedom (CCF), a food- and restaurant-industry-funded non-profit organization founded in 1996 as an advocacy group with a mission to conduct research and education on food, beverage, and lifestyle issues, challenged the "hype" about the obesity epidemic in a 2004 report and a related advertisement. The CCF is backed by considerable economic resources and had an operating budget of almost $9 billion in 2009, according to the organization's 2009 Form 990.[10] The fact that the CCF is essentially a lobbying group of the food industry, however, is discrediting and undermines its cultural authority.

Dove, a subsidiary of Unilever, has resisted the mainstream fashion idea that only excruciatingly thin women can be beautiful in its "Real Beauty" campaign. Valued at $79.32 billion in 2007, it has high levels of economic capital, although not, as measured in terms of wealth, as much as, say, Hoffman-La Roche.[11] The aesthetic and symbolic skills it deploys in its advertisement campaigns also confer considerable symbolic capital. Bariatric doctors, who have been strong proponents of a medical frame, are shown in the top left quadrant, toward the middle of the vertical access. This represents that, while they do not have as much cultural authority as the CDC, NIH, or WHO, and while bariatric medicine is not especially highly regarded within the medical field, medicine nonetheless has considerable cultural authority and is associated with high earnings (economic capital).[12] As doctors, bariatric doctors are imbued with more economic and cultural authority than the Association for Size Diversity and Health (ASDAH), which is comprised overwhelmingly of women in the less prestigious and lower-paying fields of psychology, nutrition, social work, education, and art.[13]

Thanks to the advanced degrees of its members, ASDAH has more symbolic authority as well as greater overall volume of capital, however, than fat acceptance organizations, including the National Association to Advance Fat Acceptance (NAAFA), which is also highly feminized. Fat pornography is featured in the bottom right quadrant, reflecting that it has little capital within the fat field, and, in contrast to NAAFA, higher-brow magazines, or fat acceptance blogs, its power is skewed toward economic, rather than symbolic, capital.

Illustrating unequal power relations within the fat field, in response to a question about how the fat acceptance movement is different from the Health at Every Size or HAES(sm) movement, leading fat acceptance activist, Director of Medical Advocacy for the Council on Size and Weight Discrimination, and former member of Fat Underground (FU), Lynn McAfee explains, "I think [HAES researchers] have credibility and [fat acceptance activists] don't. I think that's really it in a word."[14] McAfee says that because she does not have a medical degree, she is often dismissed out of hand: "People would say to me all the time when I come up with these studies [showing that 90 to 98 percent of people who lose weight in weight-loss diets gain it back in a year or more], 'you don't know what that means, you're not a doctor.' Well, I don't have to be a damn doctor to know what a 98 percent failure rate is."[15] McAfee admits that she is "not actually particularly that interested in [health]" and exclaims: "God, I hate science!" However, she explains that she has been drawn into debates over the health risks associated with "obesity" because, as she puts it: "People get to discriminate against us because they're just trying to help us with our health." As a result, she says that she "recognized very early on that if we are ever to succeed, we have to get a foothold in the medical world and make them understand [because] when it comes down to it, the last argument is, 'oh but it's so unhealthy for you.'"

Yet, as McAfee recognizes, people lacking in scientific credentials are more likely to be dismissed out of hand. This was made clear in in-depth interviews that I conducted with researchers. In these interviews, I asked researchers to respond to different claims, in order to see what sorts of arguments they used. In one such instance, I asked Theodore VanItallie what he thought of a statement made by a fat acceptance activist who said that reading reports on the number of excess annual deaths attributable to obesity feels, to her, like a death threat rather than as genuine concern. He replied: "When you listen to what people say, you have to think about what their qualifications are for saying it." Other obesity researchers dismissed as anecdotal fat acceptance activists' claims that their repeated dieting led to weight gain. For instance, James Hill said: "Well, you really don't have the control condition there, you really don't know what would have happened to their weight if they hadn't dieted, do you?"

Bourdieu has shown that social and cultural capital are embodied, in that they shape mannerisms, posture, and what is generally thought of as personal style. However, body size and shape can also function as a specific form of *bodily capital*.[16] For instance, boxers discipline their bodies so that they can win boxing matches, thereby converting bodily capital into economic capital. To take a different example, fashion models rent their bodily capital—in their case, corresponding to culturally specific ideas of beauty, including body shape—for economic gain. Like boxers, models cultivate their bodily capital via exercise, diet, and plastic surgery, but their bodily capital is also shaped by factors beyond their personal control, including genetics and aging.[17] More generally, in many societies, being tall, especially for men, confers status, whereas being short is discrediting. Similarly, being very thin—the proverbial 90-pound weakling—can be discrediting for men. In the contemporary United States and Europe, however, a thin, for women, and a muscularly toned, for men, body confers credibility. Hard bodies are seen as evidence of a disciplined character.[18] Thin women are more likely to "marry up" and attain a high-paying job, compared to heavier women, thereby converting bodily capital into economic capital.[19] Gender and ethnicity represent other embodied dimensions of social inequality.

In the debates over fat, fat rights activists and health at every size researchers are often dismissed as having an axe to grind if they are fat or are seen as being more credible if they are thin. For instance, science reporter and author of *Fat of the Land: Our Health Crisis and How Overweight Americans Can Help Themselves*, Michael Fumento rejects the claim that one can be fat and fit, saying that such claims give "self-deceiving obese people something to hide behind, because they can (and do) assure themselves that while, yes, they burst through the ceiling of the height-weight charts long ago, they 'feel like' or 'just know' they're in damned good condition."[20] Regardless of how many advanced degrees they have, researchers run the risk of being discredited if they themselves are fat, not only for all of the reasons that fatness is generally discrediting but also because they are perceived as being biased. For instance, when I asked an obesity researcher about Steven Blair's research showing that one can be "fit and fat," this researcher said of Blair: "He is fat, and he's been exercising a lot, but he can't lose weight. But he's had a bypass himself, and he's had a myocardial infarction.... He might have been better off with weight loss as well as fitness."

In contrast, being thin (and, for men, tall) gives researchers more credibility. For instance, Glenn Gaesser, exercise physiologist and author of *Big Fat Lies: The Truth about Your Weight and Your Health,* told me how his book agent asked him what his height and weight was.[21] When he told her that he was 6'4" and 185 pounds, she said "Oh, well that's good." When she then submitted the book to editors, she said they all wanted to know what his height and weight were. She told Gaesser that "the publisher would not have taken [the book project] if [he] was fat because it would have been viewed as almost a rationalization for being fat, [as if he had] a personal axe to grind." Indeed, Fumento laments that Gaesser's weight status gives his book authority: "Gaesser's book came out just before another fat acceptance book, Richard Klein's *Eat Fat,* and half a year before yet another, Laura Fraser's *Losing It.* But it has the potential to do much more damage because the Klein and Fraser books come across as written by fat people trying to justify their conditions rather than change them.... But Gaesser is thin!"[22]

Similarly, Linda Bacon, a professor of nutrition and author of *Health at Every Size: The Surprising Truth about Your Weight,* comments in an essay on thin privilege: "My academic credentials, my thin body, and all sorts of other privileges team up to give me a ready audience for my material, and it is much less easy for [a fat woman without academic credentials] to find a forum to have her important message heard."[23] I myself have also been told that being thin makes me more credible in my critical analysis of the dominant framing of obesity. At the 2001 NAAFA convention, NAAFA members told me that they were pleased that I was doing this research because, as a thin woman, I would be taken more seriously. A publicist at UCLA later saw fit to mention in a press release about one of my articles that I was a "petite mother of two small children." When I protested, she explained that this would reduce the likelihood that I would be "dismissed as some crazy person," and I sheepishly relented.

That a fat person is incapable of speaking objectively about weight seems to be readily accepted, while the idea that a thin person would be biased in a different but equally strong direction seems less intuitive. In other words, thinness functions as an *unmarked category*, much as whiteness or maleness operate as unmarked categories for race and gender, respectively. Just as whites are often regarded as not having race and men as not possessing gender, thin people are seen as not having body size. In each case, this obscures how dominant groups are also affected, including via privilege, by systems of inequality. In this case, it forecloses discussions of how, say, a white, middle-class, thin female obesity researcher who spends enormous amounts of time, energy, and money in maintaining her slim physique may have a bias that leads her to assume that fatness is unhealthy.

However, the extent to which having academic credentials should automatically confer authority or being fat should be discrediting is precisely part of what is at stake in the fat field. Fat rights activists and health at every size researchers underscore the fact that many obesity researchers run weight-loss clinics or receive funding from pharmaceutical companies, either directly or indirectly via the IOTF, suggesting that they cannot be objective on the topic of weight loss.[24] They argue that being fat, rather than discrediting, represents a form of personal authority, in that they have firsthand experience with weight-based stigma and living in a fat body.

POSITIONALITY AND STRONG OBJECTIVITY

Philosopher of science Sandra Harding has argued that, while the ideal of value-free, impartial, dispassionate research is supposed to eliminate all social values from research, it tends only to identify and eliminate those social values and interests that are not shared by recognized scientific experts. This has allowed, she argues, those cultural assumptions and biases that are widely shared within the scientific community—such as ideas about the inferiority of women and people of color—to shape scientific research. The influence of these ideas is especially strong and unexamined in the formulation of hypotheses and identification of research questions, which are typically considered as prior to the actual scientific test.[25] Harding advocates replacing this "weak objectivity" with "strong objectivity," in which there would be a "critical examination of historical values and interests that may be so shared within the scientific community, so invested in by the very constitution of this or that field of study, that they will not show up as a cultural bias between experimenters or between research communities."[26] One powerful way to overcome such biases is to generate knowledge from the perspective of "the systematically oppressed, exploited, and dominated, those who have fewer interests in ignorance about how the social order actually works." Taking this perspective "makes strange what had appeared familiar, which is the beginning of any scientific inquiry," says Harding.[27] Drawing on Harding's insight, one would expect those people who are categorized as obese to produce valuable and new kinds of knowledge.

Indeed, the experiences of fat women have provided the inspiration for some of the earliest work on the hazards of weight loss followed by weight regain (called weight cycling or yo-yo dieting) and on the risks associated with weight-loss surgery. Most NAAFA members can share personal stories of "yo-yo dieting." For instance, a 44-year-old administrative assistant and member of NAAFA says she "doubled [her] weight through dieting in a little over twenty years." She explains that she started off weighing 125 pounds at 5'2" but felt that she should not weigh more than 110 pounds at that height and began a series of diets, each of which led to temporary weight loss followed by even more weight gain. "I still believe that had I never dieted, I'd still be pretty close to that 125," she says. Another woman told me, through tears, how her pediatrician counseled her mother to dilute her formula at the age of four months because she was too fat. A series of enforced weight-loss diets followed, only to leave her fatter and with disordered eating. NAAFA members similarly share horror stories of the physiological and psychological damage they endured from having taken prescribed amphetamines for weight loss during adolescence, the friends who died from complications related to weight-loss surgery, or the painful side effects they and others suffered—not to mention weight regain—from weight-loss surgery.

It was in "talking to the people at NAAFA" that neuroscientist Paul Ernsberger first thought of scientifically examining the complications associated with weight-loss surgery and testing whether weight-loss diets lead to subsequent weight gain and possible health consequences.[28] Not fat himself, Ernsberger has, in his words, a "large wife." While a graduate student in the late 1970s and early 1980s, he joined NAAFA and saw many of the women members have gastric bypass surgery, then be "in and out of the hospital with complications," prompting him to research the complications associated with this surgery.[29] As a result, Ernsberger says he was made chairman of the NAAFA advisory board. Later, several NAAFA members told him how their health temporarily improved when they lost weight, but, when they gained it back, their health statistics were worse than before the surgery. Ernsberger then spoke to several physicians, who confirmed that they had seen this cycle in their patients. Reviewing the scientific literature, he found research on the topic from the 1950s and 1960s, but "then it just stopped, like it hit a brick wall," in 1972. So Ernsberger conducted his own research on the topic, finding that weight cycling leads to hypertension in animal studies.[30] In the mid-1990s, he testified against the approval of weight-loss drug Redux (part of the notorious phen-fen cocktail that ultimately was linked to heart valve failure). By Ernsberger's account, he would have never conducted the research without exposure to the experiences of women in NAAFA.

Unlike Ernsberger, Steven Blair has not been personally involved with NAAFA or other fat acceptance groups. However, he says that his own experiences as someone who is "short, fat and bald," despite running 75,000 miles over the past 35 years, informs his research. Other researchers and clinicians talk about how an experience with eating disorders led them to a health at every size approach. For instance, Bacon writes in a conference paper delivered at the 2009 NAAFA convention that "as long as it is more difficult to live in a fat body, I have to fear becoming fat. This resulted in an eating disorder I endured when I was younger, along with accompanying difficulties with food, body image and self-esteem."[31] Similarly, Joslyn Smith, who has served as vice president of the ASDAH board, as a member of the public policy committee for ASDAH, and on the diversity task force for the National Eating Disorders Association, explains that she got involved with HAES as a direct result of having struggled, despite her large body size, with symptoms of anorexia. She said that she came to a realization that if she didn't change her way of thinking, she "wouldn't survive."[32]

To the extent that the fat field is dominated by the assumption that being fat is a medical problem and public health crisis and that weight loss is the goal, those who challenge these assumptions are at a disadvantage for acquiring resources. Different researchers respond to this challenge in various ways at specific points in time. For instance, Glenn Gaesser acknowledges in an interview with me that he has emphasized weight loss as a measure of his intervention's success, in order to receive NIH funding. In contrast, neuroscientist Ernsberger says that he has had difficulty getting NIH funding for his work on yo-yo dieting, since it has to pass muster by peer reviewers who are typically "so-called experts who are running weight-loss clinics" and who reject the premise that weight cycling is harmful. He says he "can't blame them entirely, because if I was running a weight loss clinic and I believed that it was harmful to repeatedly lose and regain weight, I would have to close shop." Still, he says that "if I'd had funding, I would've been able to go a lot further" with this research. Ernsberger expresses frustration that "what's been defined as an obesity expert is somebody who treats obesity." Political scientist Joan Wolf refers to this as the "expert paradox," through which "precisely what qualifies certain individuals to serve as advisers can hinder their ability to assess the literature objectively."[33]

Some researcher-scholars are trying to change these institutional constraints.[34] For instance, U.S. nutritionist Linda Bacon recounts how, in the summer of 2009, Joslyn Smith offered training in lobbying for members of NAAFA and ASDAH. Smith, in turn, speaks of the positive reception that the group of 53 ASDAH and NAAFA members got from congressional staff members "on the Hill." In a context in which getting 15 minutes is considered a lot of time, she said numerous people got hour-long meetings. Smith, Bacon, U.S. psychologist Deb Burgard, and Australian health-promotion manager Lily O'Hara set up a meeting with "someone high up" at NIH who was overseeing grants for NIH. They explained to her how the wording of many grants excluded research that did not include weight loss as a measure of the success of the nutritional and/or exercise intervention. The ASDAH members were invited to help reword grants to make them more open-ended. Bacon comments that she is "amazed that we were able to help her to make new options."

While ASDAH members work to change the way in which body size is studied within the context of health, some scholars in the humanities, social sciences, and law, in concert with fat rights activists, are creating a new field of study around *fatness* as a form of social identity. In so doing, they are following in the footsteps of gender studies, African American studies, Chicana studies, ethnic studies, and other interdisciplinary fields of research that build on related political movements. In a foreword to *The Fat Studies Reader*, Marilyn Wann describes a fat studies approach as offering "no opposition to the simple fact of human weight diversity, but instead looks at what people and societies make of this reality."[35] The publication of *The Fat Studies Reader* in 2009 was an important watershed in the establishment of this new field. Five years earlier, Wann founded the fat studies list server and invited about 50 researchers working on weight-related topics (including me) to join. Wann already knew many activists doing work on this topic, thanks to the many talks she had been giving on college campuses for about eight years. The list membership grew over time so that, as of August 20, 2012, it had 674 members, including a mix of scholars, activists, and activist-scholars. Since then, there has been a proliferation of fat studies panels at national and regional conferences of various academic associations.

In contrast to work by scholars and clinicians that takes a health at every size approach and thus challenges obesity researchers on their own terms, fat studies as a field seeks to change the terms of the debate by placing social inequality and fat subjectivity—rather than health risk—at the heart of the analysis. Given the focus on fat subjectivity, as an important object of fat studies scholarship, being fat oneself is potentially a source of authority, rather than discrediting within this new area of study.[36] Stated differently, while devalued in the fat field as a whole, fatness is a valued form of bodily capital within this specific part of the fat field.[37]

More generally, this speaks to the way in which the internal logic of particular problem frames has independent consequences for what kinds of claims and claimants are credible. To fully understand this point, we must carefully examine the distinct logic of each of these frames. These six frames—immorality, medical, public health crisis, health at every size, beauty, and fat rights—are ideal types. In other words, actual claims about body weight often mix two or more of these frames, as we will examine at the end of this chapter. By understanding the internal logic of each of these frames, however, one sees how debates over obesity/fatness are best understood as encounters between different ways of understanding fatness.

IMMORALITY FRAME

According to what I call an immorality frame, fat is condemned as evidence of sloth and gluttony. The problem is seen as a moral one, requiring a moral remedy: namely, greater self-restraint and faith in God. The master frame is that of sin. Fatness is thus likened to other sins, such as sexual immorality. According to some accounts, the belief that fat was a sign of immorality began to spread in the late-nineteenth-century United States, firmly taking hold by the beginning of the twentieth century.[38] This represented a break from earlier periods and other places in which corpulence was appreciated as a sign of beauty and high social status. Some historians contend that this shift was largely driven by economic change. Namely, the agricultural and industrial revolutions had reduced food shortages so that fatness was no longer a reliable sign of wealth. As the poor got fatter, which they did at first in part to emulate the rich, the symbolic meaning of body size flipped, and fat came to signal *low* social status. As heft became a marker for lower prestige and status, people with greater resources had more ability and motivation to avoid the stigma of corpulence.[39]

According to other accounts, while corpulence was a valued aesthetic in Europe into the late nineteenth century, thinness (at least in women) has been associated with self-control and whiteness since early in U.S. history. In this national context, fatness has long been associated with lack of